A Stroke of Health

A Stroke of Health

The Weight is Over –
How I Learned Healthy Eating

Judith H. Swartz

With Forward and Chapter Seven
by Dr. Robert L. Galloway, III, RPh, D.C.

Library of Congress Control Number: 2009906367
ISBN: Hardcover   978-1-4415-4954-9
                 Softcover   978-1-4415-4953-2

To order additional copies of this book, contact:
Xlibris Corporation
1-888-795-4274
www.Xlibris.com
Orders@Xlibris.com
61534

Contents

Acknowledgements

Many thanks to patient friend and editor, Ruth Saler, for her work and support on this effort.

Dr. Robert Galloway's help with my husband Bob's healing and my general health has been invaluable. His contribution to this book in Chapter Seven provides expert information and guidance.

Permission to use the Food Pyramid is provided by the American Diabetes Association:

> **Copyright © 2009 American Diabetes Association**
> **From http://www.diabetes.org**
> **Reprinted with permission from *The American Diabetes Association.***

I was able to make contact with my high school friend, who provided the first photo in Chapter One of this effort. Professional photographer for many years, Bill Barley was able to schedule studio time for the cover photo while Bob and I were visiting family near Bill's studio in Columbia, S.C.

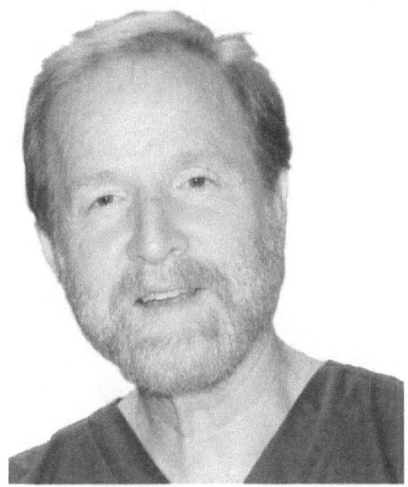

Robert L. Galloway, III, RPh, D.C. holds many degrees and certifications including Registered Pharmacist, Doctor of Chiropractic and Certified Clinical Nutritionist. As a graduate of the University of Houston College of Pharmacy, Dr. Galloway practiced as a pharmacist when a lower back injury led him to seek treatment from a local chiropractor. It was then that he discovered the health benefits of chiropractic and was compelled to pursue a career in natural health. Dr. Galloway continued to practice pharmacy while attending Palmer College of Chiropractic, where he graduated in 1981 as a Doctor of Chiropractic.

Dr. Galloway has maintained a successful chiropractic practice for 28 years in northwest Houston. His interest in nutrition has paralleled his deep commitment to improving the lives of his patients. Dr. Galloway is associated with the ACA Council on Nutrition, the American Clinical Board of Nutrition, and the International and American Associations of Clinical Nutritionists.

Dr. Galloway lives in a suburb of Houston, Texas, with his wife and three children.

Dedicated to my darling Bob and our incredible
children who are helping in this journey

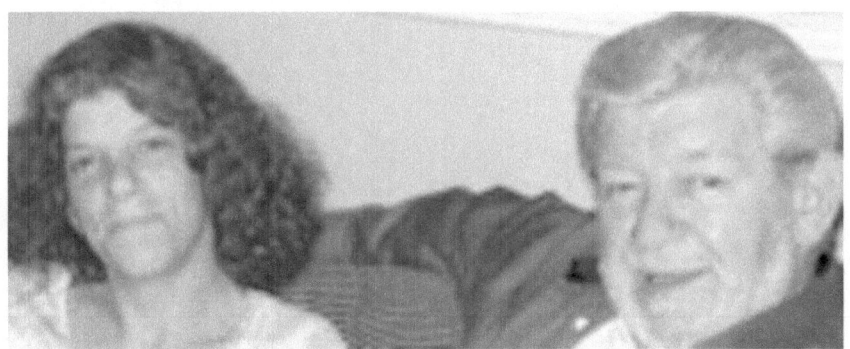

Bob and daughter Linda

Forward

The author, Judith Swartz, has given us a concise view of her voyage of discovery to better health. This is a quick read and will give the reader valuable insights into taking control of their own health. Medicine has continued to excel at emergency and life-saving interventions, but they have forgotten what health is. Judith has shown that good health is something that needs to be managed by the patients themselves. Each individual needs to be responsible for improving their own health status.

Dr. Bob Galloway

Introduction

My story is not an endorsement of anything – except "healthy eating." I only share the path to my discovery of nearly magical results after many years of riding the weight roller coaster. It's a shame that it took my husband Bob's near death to lead me to this simple truth.

I've had no medical training. My credentials are only that I've lived in a mortal body for way over 50 years – overweight for many of those. I've mothered nine children; grandmothered a few more, and am currently caring for my stroke-victim husband, who also suffers from type 2 diabetes and high blood pressure. I've always known that healthy eating is necessary for a healthy body, and that a healthy body is not a fat one. Now I know beyond any doubt that to save his life, I *must* feed Bob correctly. A healthy body will heal itself, and we *can* avoid chemicals that create other problems and compromise precious organs.

I myself have always shunned chemicals because it made no sense to me how any chemical could treat just one ailment and not affect the entire body. I have also observed many of our children ruin their bodies and brains, their very lives, with drugs and alcohol. I once asked a doctor who was offering me some drug or another, how it could possibly travel *only* to the specific area without reaching the rest of the body. He stared at me blankly. Most doctors I know, even when pressed, will only briefly explain which organs are compromised by certain drugs. No problem for them, they can continue to prescribe other drugs, providing repeat customers for other physicians, labs, hospitals and insurance providers . . . creating, in my opinion, a vicious circle that can only spiral downward.

Once during a physical exam, my physician was amazed that I had never taken female hormones. Touting the advantages, he responded to my questions about published serious side effects (like hemorrhage and death), saying proudly that they would not occur "without warning."

So, if I take these, then what?
Just see me every six months.
And if I don't take them?
Well, then you don't have to come back.

That doctor also provided me with the news that my bladder would soon fall out, and that I should have it repaired immediately. I never went back, and after 30 years it still hasn't left my body.

The only medical advice concerning weight loss that I ever received was, "Lose weight." Once while recovering from a broken ankle, one "specialist," while looking for an explanation for the ongoing pain and numbness in the ankle, shared with me, "You know what they say, you can never be too rich nor too thin." (Translation: You're too fat, lady.)

Understanding that each human body has it's own quirks, I realized I would have to figure this out – for myself, on my own. I am thankful for the information that I finally found and most especially for the caring information, guidance and treatments from Dr. Robert Galloway, who contributed the chapter on thyroid dysfunction and treatment.

If you're on a journey to jump off the weight roller coaster, I sincerely hope that you find help and inspiration in my words. Chat with me by email, *judi@judiswartz.com.*

Chapter One

My Story

Skating, swimming, walking, biking and cheerleading were everyday activities for my friends and me throughout high school. I was described as the "tall skinny girl with long hair and glasses." Before the model Twiggy made her debut, it was embarrassing to have a 19" waist, and my goal was to gain two pounds so I could weigh in at 120. Thankfully, my mother was an expert designer and seamstress, and I enjoyed a gorgeous wardrobe that would have otherwise been impossible for my family to afford.

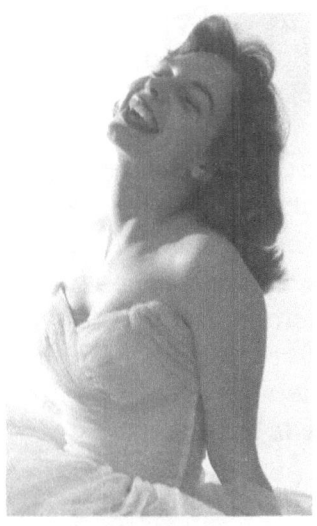

Judi at 15

Photo by Bill Barley

In my first semester of college, before marriage and babies, I quickly reached my goal of 120 pounds, plus 15 more, and I felt miserable. When I eventually remembered to omit the forbidden foods, I was once again able to don my lovely wardrobe.

A few years ago, after completing physical therapy for the smashed right ankle, I made a trip to Santa Monica. For years I had imagined myself skating from the Santa Monica Pier to Venice Beach, and my surgeon approved my quest. Aided by a friend strong enough to provide some help, I made a miserable attempt, not even getting close to the goal. Not one to give up easily, when a business trip took me there again six months ABS ("after Bob's stroke") and after I had finally shed some pounds, I reset that goal. Although my recently broken *kneecap* was now repaired, I was still experiencing enough pain to elicit caution. Believing that this was a second chance to reach my goal of skating to Venice Beach, I planned to try again, sans the helper. Unfortunately, after a long workweek, that knee was stiff and painful and I decided, much to Bob's relief, that perhaps it was not a wise idea, for all the obvious reasons.

My alternate course of action was to pile more layers on Bob's constantly cold body (he looked a bit like the "Unabomber" in his red hoodie with "Santa Monica" bolded across the front) and push him, via wheelchair, to Venice Beach and back. We made it! Daughter Linda and I shopped, Bob enjoyed a hot dog, and at least *two* of us had a great time!

My "nutrition" education took place in high school home economics class and at the dinner table. In class I remember baking biscuits, muffins and chocolate cake. At home we were encouraged to eat "a meat and two vegetables" at dinner. I was never a breakfast eater and lunch was eaten in the school cafeteria. Eating out was not within our budget, and that was BFF ("before fast food"). Desserts were limited, except on holidays, which generally included sour cream cake, pies, elegant fruitcakes and homemade ice cream.

My family maintained a list of fattening forbidden foods, including peanut butter, bread and potatoes (except on Saturday nights with steak). Carbonated sodas were not in the budget either. We drank skim milk made from powder and substituted homemade mayonnaise for store-bought. (Made with mineral oil, you ate only a very small amount lest you spend too much time in the bathroom.)

My first child was born when I was 21. In those days (don't you hate that phrase?) gaining more than 20 pounds during pregnancy was not tolerated, and the OBGYN prescribed diet pills to keep me within that range. I quickly returned to "normal," but after the birth of my second child (12-1/2 months later), "normal" eluded me. During that pregnancy, not only was I prescribed diet pills, but tranquilizers as well, to help with the stress of divorce.

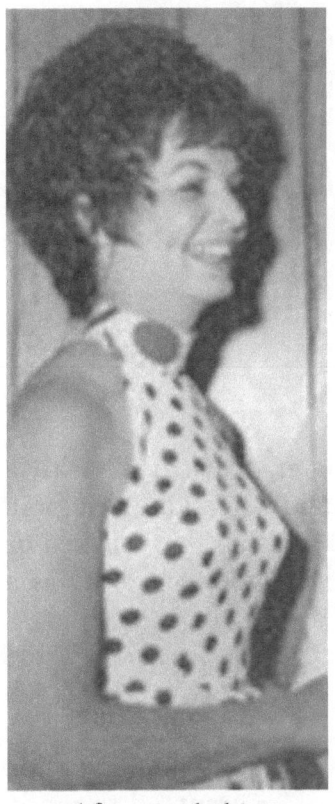

After two babies

At 22 I had left an abusive husband and was raising two children. I borrowed (size 14) clothes for my first job interview, which carved out my career path for the ensuing 10 years. Busy now with two jobs, school and parenting – with much help from my family – I was still looking for answers about healthy eating and the weight roller coaster ride intensified.

For a year I worked in an office in the morning, took some general education classes at the local university in the afternoon, and played second violin in the Charlotte Symphony in the evening. By the time I was offered full-time status at the office job, my income requirements mandated that I discontinue the college classes. Although I was constantly on the run, I was getting no real exercise whatsoever.

Someone once told me that if you ate nothing but meat, any meat cooked in any way, you would lose weight. Fueled with another prescription for diet pills, I began a diet of fried chicken and a liquid low-calorie meal replacement. It worked and I was back to in a smaller size – temporarily.

It was an up and down battle for the next 10 years.

When I met Bob, I was a size 10; but by the time we were married four years later, I was a size 14. Happier than ever, I was more relaxed and enjoying cooking for my new, much larger family. Any weight I lost – and more – returned. "You carry it well," I was told. Thank goodness my mother taught me to sew, because during the next pregnancy, without diet pills, I needed *lots* of *large* clothing – both during and after.

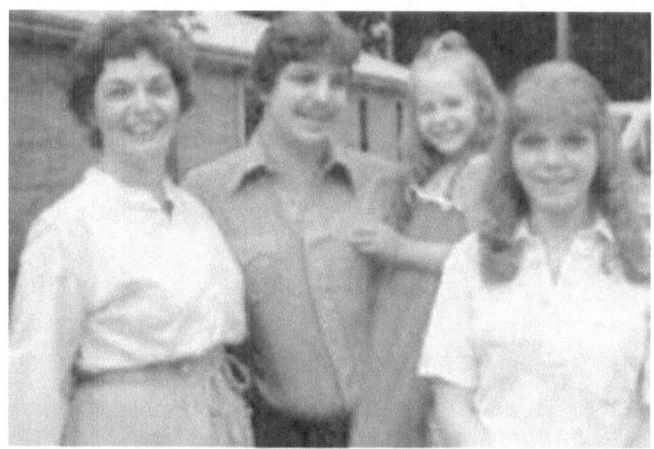

After three babies

After considerable "ballooning," six years later, I lost it all with a popular liquid diet. But I was unable to maintain when I ate real food. My search for the right way to eat provided nothing that worked or made sense. All my medical exams resulted in "you're healthy as a horse, just lose the weight."

Okay – but *how?*

In my library are copies of most of the popular eating guides, recipe books and pamphlets describing pills that are "guaranteed to work, or your money cheerfully refunded." I tried them all, and to this day, there has *never* been a refund on any of the magic pills. Prior to his stroke, Bob made the most recent of these purchases, a highly touted pill program to remove belly fat. When I complained that they would start charging our credit card every month, Bob said, "Oh, no, they

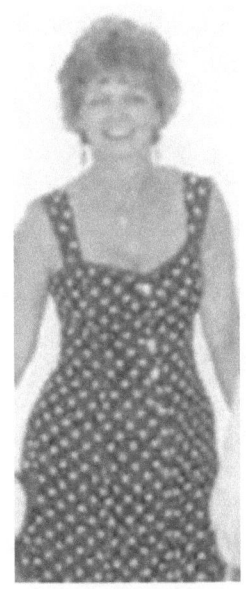

After liquid diet

said they would just send the free trial . . ." The pills didn't work and you know how that one ended!

When our last baby was seven, I returned to work, wearing my fat clothes. It was at this time that I discovered the "liquid food diet" and *that* was perfect.

Slimmer for a while, soon I was fatter than ever.

Ten years later the "packaged food diet" was the answer. Providing live radio testimonials in return for program fees and food, I eventually reached that glorious size eight – for a few minutes. I remember a wonderful moment of donning a pair of black jeans in that perfect size. But, as a famous actress once said about the high protein diet, "it works great till you eat one crouton – then it all comes back."

Once again I was not able to maintain the weight and went for yet another spin on the roller coaster – gaining even more. Up and down, regaining more after every loss, I was just about resigned to be "tons of fun" forever. Still researching the right way to eat, I observed the fat and skinny people everywhere I went. I learned several things that made no sense to me.

Skinny people drink sugared soft drinks; Fat folks drink the diet stuff. Skinny people eat everything; my fat friends pick at their food, forgoing the rice, bread and desserts (except maybe for three blueberries). Dear Erma Bombeck once wrote, " . . . only fat people eat cottage cheese." I once knew a very small person who ate only lettuce and drank scotch.

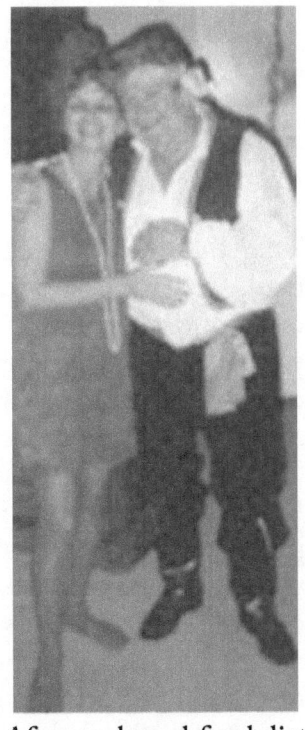

After packaged-food diet

When I felt sufficiently comfortable to pose direct questions about dietary habits, here are some of the responses I received from my personal survey:

> I choose to get my carbs from alcohol instead of eating
> food – you can't have both.
> You *must* eat six to eight meals a day
> (cook at night and carry little frozen packages with you).
> Fasting is the only thing that works.
> You can eat anything, if you wrap it in lettuce.
> Don't eat carbs.
> Don't eat protein.
> Eat only protein.
> Eat only vegetables.
> Eat only fruit and salads.
> Don't drink coffee.
> Drink coffee.
> Don't eat sugar.
> Don't eat anything white.
> Eat only a small number of calories a day.
> Eat only a large number of calories a day.
> Eat only what you crave – even if it's a piece of cake.

I was totally confused.

Then there were the card exchange programs: little folders containing cards describing food choices that you moved from one side to the other during the day. That made no sense to me either, as it is difficult enough just keeping up with my business cards. And life moves too quickly for me to look at cards every time I put something in my mouth – oops, that card has already been moved.

I observed people who live at the gym ... and those who run a marathon every month, or bicycle to three cities and back each weekend. I have problems just staying upright. Not at all graceful, the only medical problems I have ever had resulted from falling – broken ankles and toes, sprained arms, back, and neck, and broken ribs that resulted in a fractured kidney and near death. All this happened just from walking, or should I say *not* walking well. In our home gym I once fell from the treadmill, walking less than one mile per hour. The treadmill is not designed for my multi-tasking of walking and talking at the same time. Bob was on the phone to one of our children, "I have to go now, Judith just fell off the treadmill . . ." It was funny even as it happened and thankfully, nothing was broken.

A firm believer in the importance of moving the body for balance and general good health, I can't say that any one form of exercise has ever helped me lose weight. Certainly, time spent in the gym was helpful for core strength, balance and perhaps toning, but not enough for me to crave it. Since the recumbent bicycle is now part of Bob's therapy, I've considered that again for myself, knowing that backaches will disappear quickly with just a few minutes a day and some of the "fluffy" will firm.

So now you have a very brief overview of my quest. I know it's not unusual – I've watched the Oprah Show. Speaking of Oprah, that's where things started to change for me. Thanks to some great eye-opening segments from that daily information source and the writings of Gregg Braden and Dr. Wayne Dyer, I have finally learned to love my body and myself. I once heard the lovely Meryl Streep say that she was a size 14. How beautiful she is! I changed my goal. Instead of vowing to get back to the size I was in high school, if I could look *anything* like that beautiful woman, I would be happy about my figure!

Oprah's segment about the "real women" in the Dove soap commercial inspired me. I threw away the scales. Surely they were broken anyway – they just kept going up and up and up. I would weigh, cry and vow to never eat another bite – until I got hungry – so hungry, that it didn't matter what was in front of me. I was totally confused anyway, so why bother?

In truth, the scriptures have always pointed the way. The Apostle Paul wrote in Philippians 4:11-12, "I have learned to be content whatever the circumstances." I have contemplated that phrase for most of my life and only now am beginning to understand the message. I would pray, begging for help and thanking God in advance. That was part of my change – prayer without ceasing. Thank you God for my healthy body, thank you God for my healthy body . . .

Personal development has been a study for years, with success in areas of business at least. So, *why* can't I learn how to eat?

One day just last year as a young woman was eating a sandwich in my office, I asked her, "How do you do that and stay so slim?"
     She looked surprised, "What do you mean?"
     "The *bread*," I said.
     She smiled, "Bread is okay, it's good for you."
     Surely she just doesn't get it; I sighed and walked away.
     Later I asked, "Do you know how to eat?
     "Sure," she said.
     "Will you teach me?"
     "Of course, just tell me what you like to eat."

How could that possibly have anything to do with it? Obviously, she did not understand my quest for healthy eating. I had tried *that* diet too – eating whatever you crave because that's what your body needs. I know it only makes you fatter!

Just two years ago, before the last push to over 210 pounds, I avoided the camera as much as possible, hiding behind children and pets.

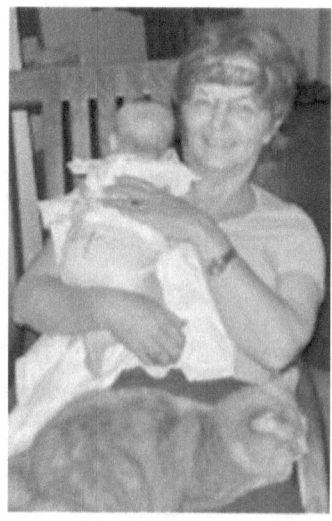

Hiding

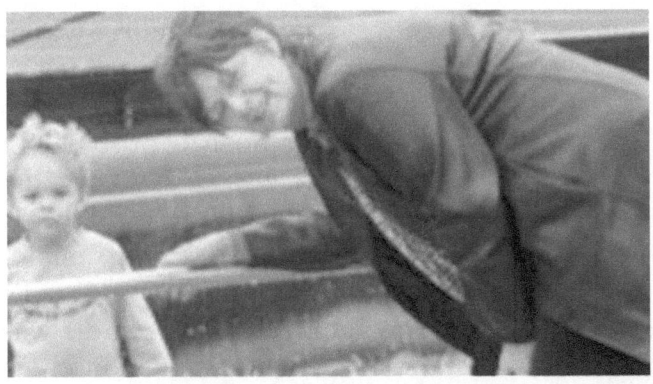

Maybe if I lean over you can't see me – look at Ben!
And it kept getting worse . . . lose one pound, gain five, six . . .

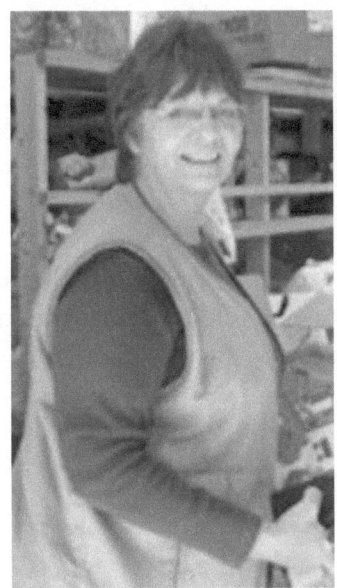

Worse

Traveling was miserable – why *do* they continue to reduce the seat size on airplanes?

And there was a strange, amazing phenomenon in my closet. Everything that hung there *shrank*.

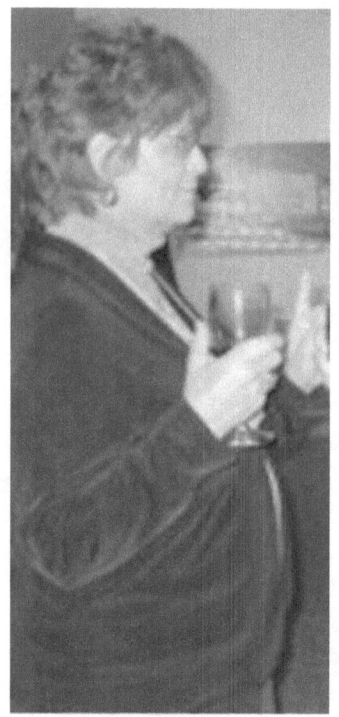

No kitten or grandchild to hide anything here

Always fairly energetic, I was now having a hard time keeping up with my peers, many of whom were half my age. That had never been a problem before. But now there was *no way* I could even begin to keep up with these children and fitness fanatics. Someone once made a remark, in public, about my weight. That person was tacky and rude, and I was certainly not the heaviest person there – and at least *I* was sober.

Once at a wedding reception, one of my son's new in-laws gushed, "Wow, you look *great*! I understand you have nine children. Wow!"

Not wanting to take unearned credit, I explained, "I only gave birth to three of them."

"Oh my," and she stepped back to look me up and down, "Well. You look *pretty* good."

And that was during one of my thinner spells.

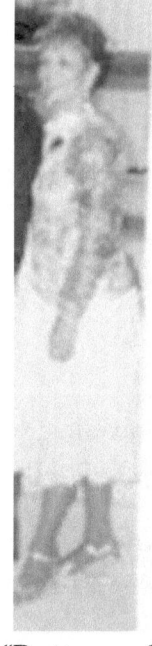

"Pretty good"

Chapter Two

Friday the 13th

Life was good. Bob and I reveled in our empty nest. We enjoyed each other, movies, sailing, travel, visits with children and grandchildren, meals out, meals in and dinner parties. We ate all the forbidden foods. When there was no wind and it was Houston-hot, we spent glorious weekends by the pool, reading, listening to music, sunning and swimming. We enjoyed light yard work, keeping our eclectic collection of pots filled with blooming plants, which is easier for me than trying to create a real garden. With busy work schedules, we were selective with social events, scheduling as much time to ourselves as possible.

The weekdays were busy, but began nicely with coffee in bed, watching the news. We took turns with the coffee making and serving, sometimes with toast or biscotti. Bob would record TV shows he thought I would enjoy, and we'd watch them (lots of Oprah) on the weekends sans commercials.

Monday through Friday at work I was dealing with very full days and some evening events that were (and still are) busy and exciting. I could never understand how Bob could accomplish so much. He managed his consulting firm, counseled clients, fed the cats, took out the trash, went to the dry cleaners/laundry, handled the swimming pool maintenance and yard work, changed the air filters and shopped for all the groceries and household supplies. He kept the cars, RV and boat maintained. We hired someone to clean the house and I was in charge of the cooking; however, Bob ate breakfast and lunch out every day, and at least a couple of times a week we went out for dinner or picked up take out. He was always looking for ways to make things easier for me.

Even with all the activity, I noticed that Bob was sleeping more, often even napping during a break at his office. We both knew he had high blood pressure and type 2 diabetes. He was seeing doctors trying to get his blood pressure at least close to the normal range. The side effects of the medications were difficult, and I think he just got tired of trying to deal with them and the poor results, and perhaps tired even of the doctors themselves.

Bob kept charts of his blood pressure and blood sugar counts, in charge of his own body as I was dealing with my weight issue. My search for healthy eating was not his goal, and I think that even today he is just beginning to understand the relationship between diet and health. Before the stroke, Bob seemed to think that as long as he took his sugar meds he could chow down a whole bag of Skittles afterward.

I would cook perceived "healthy" meals, and Bob would complain about the contents and portions, still wanting a huge bowl of ice cream enhanced with chocolate syrup and nuts every night. I would join him, perhaps for a smaller amount.

Early that fateful week, our refrigerator went on the blink. My husband was diligent, researching and shopping, and he called me to report on his findings.

It all sounded good to me; "Whatever you think," I said.
"No, you should go look and let me know what you want."
"Okay," I promised, but just never was able to get away.

Bob finally made the decision, paid for the purchase and set delivery for Monday, June 16. Always on top of everything, my husband had also scheduled a specialist to diagnose and repair a pool leak and a roofer to repair a couple of shingles.

While Bob kept the tires checked, the oil changed on all three cars and the motor home, he also kept his car washed. He handled all of our finances as well. For years I ignored his requests to learn about them, always promising to do that later. That seems to be my pattern. He had recently rebalanced the investments in our 401(k)s, and when the stock market began to plummet, we held our own.

I am often awed by some of his instincts.

Around 3:00 p.m. on that Friday the 13th, Bob called to say that he had an appointment and asked if I would leave early to meet the roofer at the house at 4:00.

Sure. I gathered the phone number of a new client and headed to my car. Weekend traffic in Houston begins just after lunch on Friday, and the normal one-hour drive 10 miles to my home could take twice that. At 3:15 I was on my cell phone at a long stoplight advising a client. The phone alerted me that Bob was calling; not unusual. I was positive that he was just calling to make certain I was en route and/ or to provide new information. Nevertheless, I quickly finished the client call and hit the speed dial for his office. Bob sounded upset (did I mention that he's a roaring Leo? He claims that he's just "passionate"), and after something I couldn't understand, I heard, " . . . I'm having a stroke . . ." and the line went dead.

Thinking that he must be pretty upset about something, I called back to see if I could calm him. This time it was very clear, "I'm *having* a stroke," he yelled in a voice that sounded very far away and strange.

Terror struck me. Looking around at the traffic, I had no doubt that I would not make the few miles to his office quickly.

Stupidly, I said, "Call 911. I'll be there in a minute."

"They're on the other line. Come now! They don't understand that my door is locked and I can't get to it." The front office was just a few feet from his desk and the door was maybe 20 feet from there. The rug burns on his knees took months to heal.

My heart was pounding. Stay calm. Stay focused. PRAY!

"I'll be right there," I promised again.

I called 911 not really expecting to talk to anyone who could help. Quickly an operator assured me that they were on the way and knew that they would have to break in to get to him. I remain thankful for the real people handling those calls! Those few minutes crawled by like hours in molasses, like a nightmare of terror, unable to move, screams with no sound.

In Bob's office parking lot were EMS vehicles and police cars – lots of flashing lights. As I approached the elevator doors, they stopped me. Calmly, serious, "You can't go up, they are working on him now."

Too stunned to argue, I waited another eternity.

On the stretcher, he was gray, clammy and soaking wet from head to toe.

"You'll be fine," I prayed as he reached for my hand, his eyes glazed.

Bob requested they take him to the hospital near our home. We were firmly told that first they would have to verify the stroke. That took seconds. Then, "For a stroke, ma'am, we need to take him to XYZ Hospital."

No questions, no arguments. "GO! I want to follow."

"Sorry, ma'am, that's not possible. You'll have to go another way."

That was one of many times I wished I had learned to use and keep in my car the GPS navigational system with the voice we named "Witch Hazel." I've been driving this city for 10 years and still had no idea how to get to XYZ Hospital, though I do remember being lost in that area several times.

One of the police officers, now visibly shaken, provided directions for avoiding some of the traffic. Calm, be calm, I willed myself. Write this down. A sticky note with the driving directions was now on my windshield.

Middle of June. Hot – Houston hot. Humid. I was enveloped in terror that I could have never imagined. Praying for God's traveling mercies and Bob's life, I somehow made it to the address scribbled on the paper. The front entrance touted valet parking. Entering quickly and forcing myself to breathe, I requested directions to the emergency room. It was at least two blocks away, but the walk was thankfully inside the building, allowing me a few minutes of air conditioning.

Where is my husband, Bob Swartz?

Hospital personnel were polite but had no idea to whom I was referring. Stepping behind their desk, I picked up the phone and dialed 911. Politely, I was referred to another number that automatically put me on hold. It did not take too long to learn that he was at a *different* XYZ Hospital. With a pounding heart, I made my way back to the car (they graciously waived the $20 fee).

The correct XYZ Hospital had easy access to the emergency room and I stopped by the entrance. Later I picked up a hospital phone, explaining about my haphazard parking. "Not a problem, we'll send someone to pick it up and park for you."

It was like a scene from a dramatic movie. Dedicated, trained, kind doctors, nurses, and technicians were caring for my Bob. I must write about those next few months in detail – but in another place.

After Bob was moved from the ICU, we were provided with loads of information, much of it conflicting and confusing. Diets prescribed by the specialists did not appear on the meal trays. Since it was imperative that a family member be present at all times, we made notes, asked questions, made more notes and studied together in the late evenings, trying to prepare for a homecoming, if there was to be one. I clearly understood that Bob's life depended on healthy eating, and I needed to learn exactly what that meant.

Daughter Linda called from Atlanta to say that she was moving in with us to help care for her dad. What a blessing! I had been struggling with how I could continue working and still provide loving care for Bob by myself. Linda quickly learned her dad's medications and continues to manage those every day. She helps with his personal needs, plays cards with him, shares the mutual interest in NASCAR racing, and somehow manages to keep our home spotless and orderly. Linda takes over when I depart each morning and shares emergencies when they arise. It's such a comfort for us both to have a daughter and friend at home with us. Without her help, we would never have been able to travel to Santa Monica or make many of our outings. Linda and I together research and apply our new-found knowledge to Bob's diet and exercise regime.

We recently embarked on the adventure of driving from Houston to Charlotte, N.C. for a family gathering. Linda and I high-five each other as we work together to streamline the tasks of moving Bob safely from car to chair, chair to car, car to chair . . . and hefting the chair in and out of the trunk, attempting to escape injury to ourselves. Perhaps that's my "exercise program."

Chapter Three

Discovery

The Food Pyramid

I discovered the Food Pyramid provided by the American Diabetes Association (The First Step in Diabetes Meal Planning) somewhere within all the books, notes and information provided by the hospital. It seemed simple enough on the surface, but became quite complicated in its detail. And it certainly did not correlate to the meals the hospital was feeding my husband. My instincts told me that this chart would be key to Bob's recovery.

Now taped to the door of my lovely new refrigerator next to the blood sugar guidelines, I started at the top of the Pyramid. Not only did I now have a road map for healthy eating, I also was armed with all the right equipment for monitoring my Bob's sugar level and blood pressure.

I believed that his life depended on me.

It was then that I determined that Bob and I would eat *everything* on the list – *every day*.

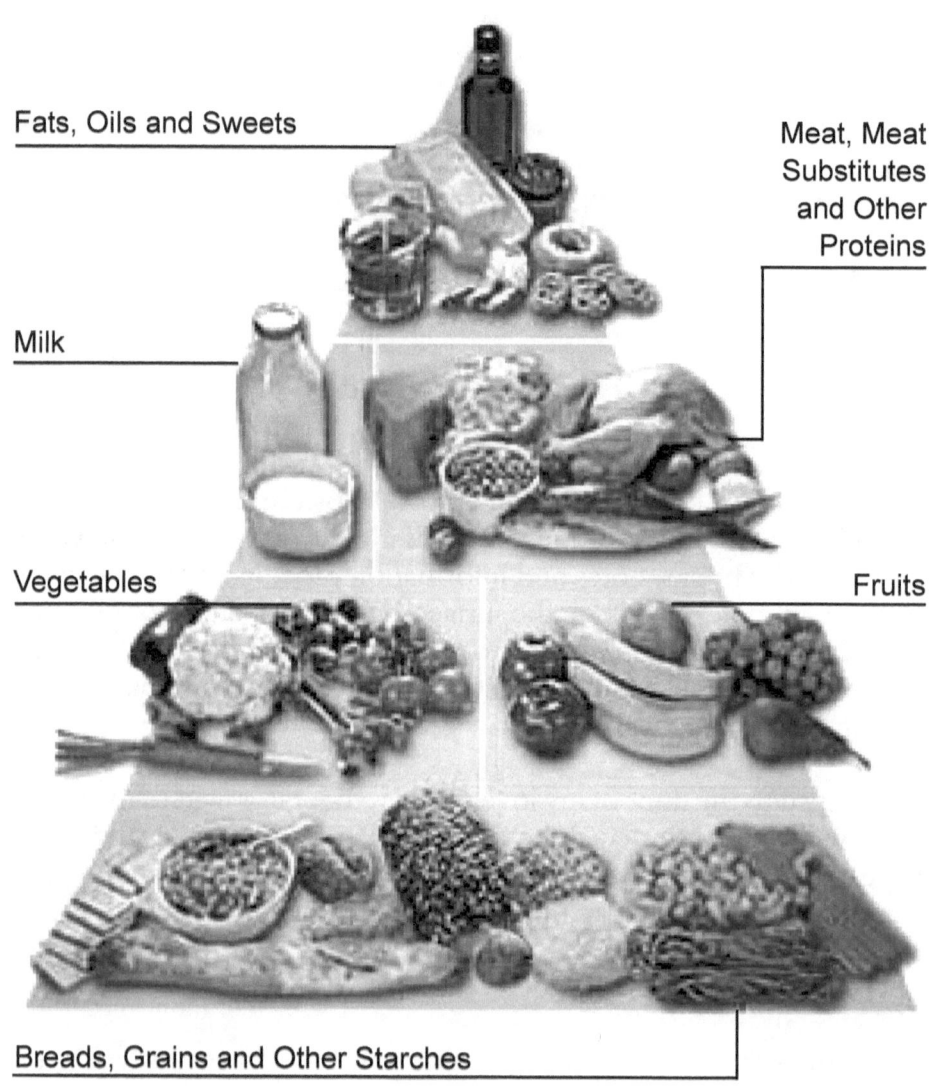

Fats, Oils and Sweets

Meat, Meat Substitutes and Other Proteins

Milk

Vegetables

Fruits

Breads, Grains and Other Starches

Food Pyramid

The Diabetes Food Pyramid divides food into six groups. These groups or sections on the Pyramid vary in size. The largest group – grains, beans, and starchy vegetables – is on the bottom. This means that you should eat more servings of grains, beans, and starchy vegetables than of any of the other foods. The smallest group – fats, sweets, and alcohol – is at the top of the Pyramid. This tells you to eat very few servings from these food groups.

On April 19, 2005 the United States Department of Agriculture (USDA) released a new food guidance system replacing the former Food Guide Pyramid. The new system, called "My Pyramid," provides a set of tools based on caloric requirements to help Americans make healthy food choices.

The Diabetes Pyramid provides a range of servings. If you follow the minimum number of servings in each group, you would eat about 1600 calories and if you eat at the upper end of the range, it would be about 2800 calories. Most women would eat at the lower end of the range and many men would eat in the middle to high end of the range if they are very active. The exact number of servings you need depends on your diabetes goals, calorie and nutrition needs, your lifestyle, and the foods you like to eat. Divide the number of servings you should eat among the meals and snacks you eat each day.

The Diabetes Food Pyramid is a little different than the USDA Food Guide Pyramid because it groups foods based on their carbohydrate and protein content instead of their classification as a food. To have about the same carbohydrate content in each serving, the portion sizes are a little different too. For example: you will find potatoes and other starchy vegetables in the grains, beans and starchy vegetables group instead of the vegetables group. Cheese is in the meat group instead of the milk group. A serving of pasta or rice is 1/3 cup in the Diabetes Food Pyramid and ½ cup in the USDA pyramid. Fruit juice is ½ cup in the Diabetes Food Pyramid and ¾ cup in the USDA pyramid. This difference is to make the carbohydrate about the same in all the servings listed.

Following is a description of each group and the recommended range of servings of each group.

Grains and Starches

At the base of the pyramid are bread, cereal, rice, and pasta. These foods contain mostly *carbohydrates*. The foods in this group are made mostly of grains, such as wheat, rye, and oats. Starchy vegetables like potatoes, peas, and corn also belong to this group, along with dry beans such as black eyed peas and pinto beans. Starchy vegetables and beans are in this group because they have about as much carbohydrate in one serving as a slice of bread. So, you should count them as carbohydrates for your meal plan.

Choose 6-11 servings per day. Remember, not many people would eat the maximum number of servings. Most people are toward the lower end of the range.

Serving sizes are:
  1 slice of bread
  ¼ of a bagel (1 ounce)
  ½ an English muffin or pita bread
  1, 6 inch tortilla
  ¾ cup dry cereal
  ½ cup cooked cereal
  ½ cup potato, yam, peas, corn, or cooked beans
  1 cup winter squash
  1/3 cup of rice or pasta

Vegetables

All vegetables are naturally low in fat and good choices to include often in your meals or have them as a low calorie snack. Vegetables are full of vitamins, minerals and fiber. This group includes spinach, chicory, sorrel, Swiss chard, broccoli, cabbage, bok choy, brussels sprouts, cauliflower, and kale, carrots, tomatoes, cucumbers, and lettuce. Starchy vegetables such as potatoes, corn, peas, and lima beans are counted in the starch and grain group for diabetes meal planning.

Choose at least 3-5 servings per day.

A serving is:
> 1 cup raw
> ½ cup cooked

Fruit

The next layer of the Pyramid is fruits, which also contain carbohydrates. They have plenty of vitamins, minerals, and fiber. This group includes blackberries, cantaloupe, strawberries, oranges, apples, bananas, peaches, pears, apricots, and grapes.

Choose 2-4 servings per day

A serving is:
> ½ cup canned fruit
> 1 small fresh fruit
> 2 tbs dried fruit
> 1 cup of melon or raspberries
> 1 ¼ cup of whole strawberries

Milk

Milk products contain a lot of protein and calcium as well as many other vitamins. Choose non-fat or low-fat dairy products for the great taste and nutrition without the saturated fat.

Choose 2-3 servings per day

A serving is:
> 1 cup non-fat or low-fat milk
> 1 cup of yogurt

Meat and Meat Substitutes

The meat group includes beef, chicken, turkey, fish, eggs, tofu, dried beans, cheese, cottage cheese and peanut butter. Meat and meat substitutes are great sources of protein and many vitamins and minerals.

Choose from lean meats, poultry and fish and cut all the visible fat off meat. Keep your portion sizes small. Three ounces is about the size of a deck of cards. You only need 4-6 ounces for the whole day

Choose 4-6 oz per day divided between meals

Equal to 1 oz of meat:
    ¼ cup cottage cheese
    1 egg
    1 Tbsp peanut butter
    ½ cup tofu

Fats, Oils and Sweets

Things like potato chips, candy, cookies, cakes, crackers, and fried foods contain a lot of fat or sugar. They aren't as nutritious as vegetables or grains. Keep your servings small and save them for a special treat!

Serving sizes include:
    ½ cup ice cream
    1 small cupcake or muffin
    2 small cookies

Chapter Four

Lifestyle Changes

Our daughter, Marye, and her children Elliott (five) and Piper (two) drove to Houston from San Antonio the day after Bob's stroke. Marye lovingly took over the household duties, including meal preparation, for which she has a great talent. The grandchildren provided much needed laughter, joy, and lots of love.

Daughter Niki set up files, made notes, and taught me how to pay the bills online. "It will probably take you a couple months to get a handle on this," she said as she guided me through our finances. When it was necessary for her to return to Oregon, she assured me that she would always be available to help by phone or email.

The stroke and the drugs took their toll on Bob, and while in the hospital he frequently had no idea where he was. He seemed confused and groggy, but amazingly, he could always provide passwords and other vital information that I sorely needed. My primary goal was to handle things without causing him additional stress. "Just concentrate on getting better, I can handle this," I promised, still wondering exactly how I would do that.

For days after that fateful Friday, I was unable to swallow any solid food. Leaving the hospital most evenings as children, family and friends stood guard in Bob's room, I would call home to let Marye know that I was on the way and provide updates on Dad. Frightened and exhausted, I looked forward to the quiet late evening conversations by the pool with my children.

The abundance of strength, love and support that was heaped on me continues to amaze me.

"Are you hungry, Mom?"
"No."

To the computer I would go, to catch up on unfinished work that I had started at the hospital. Marye would bring me a beautiful plate of steamed vegetables on rice or a cool, crunchy salad with one of her delightful dressings. Odd, I thought, that this tastes so good!

A light started to come on – well, a flicker perhaps.

During those first two months, I began to notice that my clothes were getting looser. In fact, I found that I could now wear some of the suits that had mysteriously shrunk while hanging in my closet. It was a fleeting thought.

Niki made three trips from Oregon, two with our grandson, Benjamin Franklin, to help with Bob's business and provide love for us all. She introduced me to healthy meals that were tasty, and I found myself eating things that I had previously considered forbidden – beans, for example.

Soon after Bob came home in mid-August, it was time for Marye to return due to Elliott's school schedule. On my own now, I followed her examples for meal preparations using the Food Pyramid as my guide.

Chapter Five

The Stroke of Health

Fats, Oils and Sweets

The Pyramid that was included in my information reads: *Fats, Sweets and Alcohol* – servings 0-3 with each meal. It instructed, "When you do eat these make them part of your food plan. Don't eat them as extras. Limit sweets to 1 serving with 15 grams of carbohydrates." Another version suggests limiting desserts servings to 2-3 times a week. That makes the planning flexible and easy!

Alcohol

Bob generally prefers no alcohol and I enjoy a glass of wine only occasionally. Recently Linda and I panicked over what I perceived was a dramatic plunge in Bob's blood pressure. The nurse for his primary care physician said, "Well, isn't that what you've been trying to achieve?" So focused on *high* numbers, I didn't remember *normal* – and he was there, temporarily.

I calmed down a bit and Bob said with a twinkle in his good eye and a crooked smile, "Can I have pizza and beer for dinner?"
"You bet!" I promised, "After your vegetable juice."

Fats

It's been easy to learn tasty meal preparations with little or no fat. A dash of sesame oil is a wonderful flavor enhancer and I use a small amount of EVOO (that's Rachel Ray speak for extra virgin olive oil) or butter, which I prefer to margarine, in Bob's food preparations. Adding ½ – 1 teaspoon of butter to my oatmeal, unless it goes on bread, is my choice.

This is easy. A small amount of fat like butter, olive oil or avocado in each meal for healthy choices.

Sweets – We can eat desserts!

Bob can still have ice cream occasionally. We enjoy Blue Bell Vanilla, with no sugar. 1/3 cup with a couple of sugar-free cookies (we love the Murray brands) is a nice treat from time to time. It's interesting that when I follow the Pyramid guidelines, the craving for sweets disappears. This was a huge change for me. A small piece of sugar-free chocolate is quite satisfying. Bob still mentions his favorite Skittles, but seems quite satisfied with the new treats. There are many excellent options, but our favorites are the wonderful Sugar Free selections made by Russell Stover. Bob loves the Pecan Delight or Caramel (the Coconut ones are for me), and one or two occasionally cause no problems with his blood sugar. Hoo-*Ray*!

Another thing I observed is that by preparing a variety of foods, the habits have disappeared and infrequent snacks now consist of a small serving of exquisite cheese with a few healthy whole-grain, sugar-free crackers, or popcorn or pretzels (in accordance with the allowances for dairy and bread). I recently attempted to eat a piece of apple pie and was amazed that it just didn't taste very good. Linda keeps sugar-free Jell-O and chocolate pudding in the refrigerator. Some bakeries and grocery stores provide sugar-free products. Although it's important to read the labels carefully, you'll find some nice options for sweets or desserts. A recent cherry pie was one of those for us. Planning to serve a small piece after lunch, I just reduced the fruit servings in the morning smoothie and omitted the bread serving with the lunch. No one noticed. A family favorite cobbler recipe will have to be revised, as it is just too terribly sweet. Bottom line for me is that sweets are just not a big deal anymore.

Milk 2 – 3 servings per day

I can drink *milk*! Having avoided milk for so many years, this is a real treat. We use low-fat milk on oatmeal, and each morning I make a fruit smoothie with plain low-fat yogurt (White Mountain purchased in large containers until I learn how to make my own). It's healthy and delicious, and it helps meet the requirements for two to three servings per day. See Smoothie recipe under *Fruits*.

Alternatives to milk are many. Ice cream with no sugar added, a small milk shake or yogurt (with or without fruit, or add some granola). I can drink a glass of milk or use the serving as sour cream in one of my easy favorites – Rolled Chicken Breasts.

Meat and Meat Substitutes – 4-6 oz per day

Substitutes? That sounds awful! I read on, delighted and amazed to see that there were no more "forbidden foods." The Food Pyramid provided easy instructions and the results were tasty. I've learned that *the protein at each meal* is key for us! One egg and/or a couple of slices of turkey bacon at breakfast, meat and cheese rolls or a sandwich with spinach or lettuce on multi-gain or potato bread make good use of the guidelines provided in the Pyramid. Now Bob's blood sugar readings are consistently in the "good" range, eliminating the need for insulin.

We've reduced our consumption of beef in favor of ground turkey and fish. I've discovered lots of delicious fish options including tilapia, halibut and salmon. A sauce prepared with a small amount of butter, lemon juice and capers really dresses up the flavors. Burgers made with seasoned ground turkey now taste better to me than beef.

Peanut butter on fiber bread (see pg. 46), crackers (0 sugar grams is best – not hard to find and are very tasty) and cheese, nuts and sardines make good snacks. Tuna salad is also good, but it still reminds me of the old diet days. Use your "fat" serving by including mayonnaise, and if in a sandwich, toast the bread and add fresh spinach. Canned salmon or leftover ham makes a wonderful salad, and an ounce is a good afternoon snack. There are so many delicious options when you can eat *everything*!

Some of my favorite easy cook-ahead recipes include Stew (beef, chicken, whatever you like), Salmon, Cod or Tilapia with Marye's Butter Sauce, Rolled Chicken Breast, Meatloaf and Quick Chicken Soup.

Hamburgers have taken on new meaning. At least once a month I experience urgent cravings for these guys, most often made of ground turkey seasoned with herbs, onions and garlic and served with roasted fingerling potatoes or sweet potatoes. I prepare extras on whole-wheat buns, wrap them in foil and pop them in the freezer.

Chili, soups and stews are a terrific way to make sure the meat and meat substitute requirements are met. Peas and corn are Bob's favorites, and now I know they are not only okay, but also required as starchy vegetables! Bob is a happy camper when I dish up his favorite meal of Meatloaf (see Recipes), mashed white potatoes or yams, and corn or peas. A meatloaf sandwich the next day is a fantastic lunch, and the veggie requirements will be met in the veggie juice before dinner.

Snacks are a cinch; simply refer to the Pyramid list. "Just tell me what you like to eat." *Now, I get it!*

Vegetables – A minimum of 3-5 servings per day

A minimum of 3-5 servings – that's a *lot* of veggies! Another of my personal surveys reveals that most humans don't eat nearly as many vegetables as the Pyramid recommends. We have our favorites, but *every* day?

Steamers are good, but even a variety of veggies gets a bit boring day in and day out – and it reminds me of my mother's "meat and two vegetables at each meal" philosophy. Salads are nice, but one every day doesn't come close to meeting the required amount. We all love fresh raw veggies, but *five servings a day*? A couple of carrot sticks at a party are tolerable, but that is nowhere near enough. How will I do this?

How often do you prepare red beets? Or mustard greens? Or turnips? Squash? Fresh green beans? I like beets; they're very healthy, but in the past I probably prepared them about once every 18 months. Greens are okay, maybe once or twice a year (the Southern New Year's meal is one of those events). And if you grew up in the South, they are difficult to eat without lots of bacon grease! Spinach is nice and easy to prepare quickly: wilted with a dash of sesame oil, sesame seeds, salt and pepper to taste under a serving of salmon – but NOT every day! How *will* I do this?

Steamed or sautéed fresh vegetables are okay a couple of times a week, but Bob and Linda are not fans of some of the things I like – zucchini, snow peas, etc. I've never met anyone who managed to eat enough raw vegetables as outlined in the Pyramid, and I knew that fresh or frozen were the healthiest. I *will* figure this out!

The serving suggestions provided a clue. The only way I could envision getting that many vegetables in Bob's body each day was to prepare vegetable juice.

I retrieved the juicer from the pantry and ordered at least half a dozen used books from Amazon.com, reading as fast as possible. *This* would be my solution. Now nearly every day before dinner, and based on Bob's meals for the day and his blood sugar readings, I prepare a small pitcher of juice for the three of us to share.

Basic Vegetable Juice Recipe

One small beet with all the stems and leaves
5-6 carrots (Marye says that if the carrots are not organically grown, you should remove the top and bottom)
4-6 stalks of celery
Greens – any combination of parsley, cilantro, spinach, kale and/or lettuce (Linda and Bob refuse to eat any of these, but they love the juice)
One small apple, or half of a med/large apple (remember the serving instructions for fruits)

We've experimented with radishes, mustard greens and leeks and quickly found that a very small amount of those provides a real *kick* to your drink. I now use the leeks in preparing stews and soups instead. For the juicing, we prefer kale and spinach to mustard greens. I have never eaten so many green leafies, but now look forward to the evening veggie cocktail. If a "minimum of 3-5 servings" is good, then as in most of my goal setting, I push that a bit to 5 servings or more.

Preparation becomes easier with daily routine, and I've learned to appreciate the beauty of a tray piled high with fresh vegetables quickly transforming into a colorful, healthy and tasty juice.

Initially, we all thought the drink tasted like dirt. I preferred to call it "earthy." But soon we all began to look forward to that clean taste. Juicing is a sure-fire way to include all the requirements of this important group each and every day. Observing my flatter belly and reduced "muffin top," I'm encouraged to continue this ritual! We've also observed that Bob's blood pressure and blood sugar numbers remain in the "good" range and he has *no* belly fat!

Note: It dawned on me that by juicing, I was removing the all-important fiber. One of my books includes a recipe that gave me an idea – make bread from the usually discarded vegetable pulp! Not only healthy, the bread is surprisingly tasty.

Judi's Fiber Bread

1 cup pulp from whatever you've juiced
⅓ cup oil (safflower or canola)
½ cup honey
½ – ¾ cup chopped dried fruit (I like apricots)
½ cup nuts (I like walnuts)
1 – q cup whole-wheat pastry flour
¼ tsp. salt
½ tsp. cinnamon
⅛ tsp. nutmeg
1 – 2 tsp. baking soda

Mix all ingredients in a food processor and pour in lightly oiled (or use baking spray) loaf pan. Bake at 350 degrees for 45-60 minutes or until toothpick inserted in the center comes out clean. Turn out onto a wire rack to cool. Yield: One loaf. Multiply the recipe and store extras in refrigerator or freezer. I've been making several loaves at a time, one for the fridge and two for the freezer. Slice and serve warm, cold or toasted. Optional: spread with butter, jelly, peanut butter or cream cheese. Watch your servings – remember, it's *fiber* bread.

Other vegetables that are working for us are Spinach Salad, Marye's Tomato Salad, Marye's Caesar Salad, Steamed Spinach and Steamed Zucchini, which is a great substitute for pasta under spaghetti sauce (see Recipes).

Grains, Beans and Starchy Vegetables – 6-11 servings per day (2-4 servings per meal)

I have a personal requirement to consume foods previously considered forbidden for weight loss; the things I *love* to eat. Another Hoo-*RAY!* Beans are nutritious, high in fiber and make wonderful soups. Pasta can be added to leftover soup to easily provide variety while meeting the requirements of my goal to eat *everything* on the Pyramid, every day. Thinking that there might be a catch here, I examined the labels. Most of these foods contain little or no fat or sugar! Whole-wheat flour is easy to find and there are *lots* of alternatives to regular white flour, allowing for interesting and creative options.

Now I understand why mashed potatoes and gravy were piled on the hospital trays twice a day, but in the spirit of variety – a small serving of Jasmine or brown rice is a nice complement to many meals. Not a huge fan of rice, Bob does like beans and rice occasionally. (Seeing results of healthy weight loss, no insulin and fewer pills to lower blood pressure has made an impression.) I *love* to prepare Quinoa, red is my favorite, plain or with nearly anything you like – raisins and nuts, garlic and herbs, sautéed vegetables. Recipes are usually included on the package.

Meeting the requirement for grains and starchy vegetables is a pleasure for me. Snacks are no longer omitted, and by eating everything on the Pyramid, a small serving of anything is often more than enough – amazing!

I recently made a discovery that I believe is relevant to grains. Judi's Cookies is a family favorite recipe that probably contains *way* too much sugar for healthy eating. I recently revised it with substitutions for most of the sugar, and not knowing how to determine the sugar grams per cookie, we experimented. First, I checked Bob's sugar level and gave him a cookie, rechecking the level 30 minutes later. The number was lower so I gave him another, rechecking that all-important number and then again in two hours. The sugar level dropped again. I've done that several times and the results are always the same. My only explanation for that is the high fiber content (from nuts and oatmeal) of these delicious cookies (see Recipes).

Marye makes wonderful poached eggs on crispy toasted English Muffins, sometimes adding a small amount of cheese and/or Canadian bacon. A family favorite is a variation of Bob's Grandmother's Potato Pancakes served with homemade cooked apples and sour cream.

Cereal box reading provides good information when choosing better nutritional options. My rule is to omit products that contain ingredients that sound like chemicals. Steel cut oatmeal served with a few banana slices, one chopped date and ½ cup milk is good for Bob and works for me without the bananas and date, as I prefer a small amount of brown sugar and granola.

Corn tortillas wrapped around eggs scrambled with turkey sausage make a good weekend brunch. Served after a fruit smoothie, you're on your way down the Pyramid.

The frozen food section at the grocery store is chock full of easy healthy varieties, whole grain waffles for example. Toasted and served with sugar-free jelly or jam is one way to get the grains for a meal. By serving the smoothie first and preparing an egg to go along with it, we're eating right and the rewards are many: energy, health and weight loss/management. The small amount of protein at each meal makes a major difference.

Chapter Six

Bonus

It started during the two months Bob was in the hospital. I was walking – walking a *lot*. The cane I was using for extra support for the recovering kneecap was getting in the way. I was schlepping a briefcase and laptop for work, my purse and luggage containing changes of clothes, not knowing what new complication might keep me at the hospital; clean clothes and extra covers for Bob, plus any books on CD, movies, etc. that might calm him. I brought instant oatmeal and fruit for the days that the tray was wrong or didn't appear. I brought snacks, along with vitamin supplements like B-12, aloe vera juice, ginger tea and cranberry capsules, all which seemed to be against the law in the traditional medical world. When Bob could be out of bed, I'd provide tours of the huge complex from the emergency room to ICU, the cafeterias, and shops – anything to bolster his spirits.

When Niki or Marye were with me, they would pile me in a wheelchair for a break from the long hot treks and relief for the recovering kneecap. Niki introduced me to the Chipotle Restaurant where you can customize your order to be quite healthy. There was a delightful coffee shop next door, and on a couple of very hot evenings I slipped away for a frozen margarita at Chipotle, my fully charged cell phone tucked into my bra. If I remember correctly, having his cell phone was Bob's first request in ICU – his security and constant link to me via speed dialing.

Since I was working full time, my clothes were professional each day. I began to trip on my slacks. What is that? Then I noticed that I was tugging at the waistbands, which were drooping. Did the elastic break? I don't have time to sew or shop. Wait! I'm getting smaller. That's odd. I began to dig through the why-don't-you-just-donate-them clothes and found some lovely suits that had not been worn in years. They fit! Then *they* became loose and then, too big. By the time Bob came home, I knew that I could fall again – this time on my baggy slacks. I didn't want to try to explain that in the emergency room, and I certainly didn't have time for another surgery and the climb back. So I went shopping – quickly at my favorite Marshall's.

Thinking that perhaps I *might* be able to wear size 14's, I began choosing some basic colors. They looked pretty big; maybe I'll get a couple pair of 12's. Embarrassed that someone might see me try to get into those, I just took them home where they hung in my closet for few days while I gathered the nerve to try them. While preparing for disappointment, when the time came, to my amazement, they *all* fit nicely!

In planning for a business trip in January, my goal this year was to wear a size 14 (a major improvement on the 14 and 16 Women's sizes and XL, one size fits most). What a bonus for me – to wear anything with a tag proclaiming size 12!

Grandson Elliott seemed to notice first. One Saturday while Bob was still in the hospital (so I know it was before August 18), as I headed out to the pool for a few moments with the children, Elliott stopped me and exclaimed, "Grandma, you look great!" Children are too honest to make up something like that. It was my stamp of approval, lifting my spirits to new heights.

Many of my associates thought that the stress of Bob's stroke was taking an unhealthy toll and often asked, "Are you okay?" The days were long and busy, so I combined brief shopping trips with the hospital complex outings for Bob and slowly found that my new size allowed me some welcomed fashion changes. Long jackets, flowing scarves and big shirts attempting to cover rolls of fat were being discarded and replaced with updated styles. I even dug out belts that I thought had been tossed (they shrank too), and now I had to punch new holes in the ones that were too big. Even my shoes became looser. Fitted shirts are now tucked in and I don't have to unzip my pants for the drive home! Many nights I don't even change clothes until after dinner. Previously, ripping off my tight clothing and jumping into a huge men's tee shirt was a near emergency upon arriving home.

The incredible shrinking closet has now reversed. Everything hanging there now *expands*. I can wash new jeans and as never before, put them in the dryer! They are still loose! Another recent phenomenon is that my car seems enormous. It's necessary now to raise the seat since I seem to be sitting several inches lower. And there's plenty of room for my purse. I am amazed that a regular bath towel now covers me and wraps without falling off!

As you may have guessed, by now the size 12's are swallowing me and I've moved comfortably into 10's, which are getting looser each day. A recent purchase of size 8 black jeans reminded me of a few minutes after the "packaged food" diet when I struggled into a gift from my daughters – size 8 black jeans. I don't remember wearing them more than twice since I was not able to maintain the weight loss. As I suspected, it's much easier to find a selection of styles and colors in smaller sizes. Double bonus: I recently wore my official Texas Cowboy boots with my new jeans. A Valentine gift from Bob over 30 years ago, my excuse for not wearing them recently was the smashed ankle. But when my shoes started feeling loose, it occurred to me that just *maybe* I could wear those boots. I was correct!

During the Christmas holidays, my daughters braved the after-holiday sales and Niki shopped for my new wardrobe of underwear, replacing some of the "industrial strength" items with prettier versions in smaller sizes that further enhance my new attitude. Several of the newer slacks, blouses and jackets purchased (before the Pyramid) have been altered, and dressing for work each day is actually fun!

While in physical therapy for my knee and back, Dr. Bob Galloway would answer questions and render guidance for my Bob's healing. He fulfilled his promise to help with Bob's agitation and general grumpiness by testing and providing supplements needed to allow the the body to heal itself. In the process, he inquired about Bob's thyroid function.

I had no idea. They promised to test it in the hospital, but if they did, I never received a report.

I realize my own thyroid is probably not functioning properly; the medical tests and treatments are surrounded by controversy. Perhaps a little knowledge is a dangerous thing, but my very limited understanding of hormones and treatments completely deters me from traditional drug therapy. Although the local alternative doctor is rather expensive, Bob and I had agreed early last year that I was worth the expense and should make an appointment. That was BBS (before Bob's stroke) and now the time and energy, more so than the money, were just not there.

Dr. Bob asked a few questions and gave me a test, explaining that most people today don't have enough iodine. He said, "Paint the inside of his wrist with iodine and tell me how long it takes to disappear. Next, take Bob's temperature *before* he gets out of bed every day for five days and report back to me." I followed his instructions for Bob *and* myself, delivering the results the following week.

The kind doctor explained about the lack of iodine, the history of salt – with and without iodine – and prescribed different amounts of supplements for Bob and me to enhance thyroid function. He later reminded me that this treatment would not last forever, that we were correcting a problem, and it is possible to overdose on iodine. That's good to know. I was reminded that a little knowledge can be dangerous and trusted professional guidance is vital.

It is difficult to weigh Bob since standing is difficult for him and I have not yet replaced the scales. So I didn't know his weight until just recently. I do know that he no longer has a belly and gets lost in his old clothes.

For me, it was the icing on the cake. Coupled with healthy eating, activating my thyroid has made the ongoing weight loss dramatic. And since weight loss was not even my goal, the time has not seemed long – in all, eight months and the weight is still dropping. My energy level has improved, even though I do get tired a maybe a little cranky after a non-stop 16-hour day. I'm not skinny and I have no goal to reach my childhood size, but for the first time in years I feel *normal* and have no urge to cry when I get dressed or look in the mirror. Recently someone asked if Linda and I were sisters.

I've found renewed interest in the recumbent bike and treadmill previously utilized to dry beach towels and as a playground for the grandchildren. I'm swimming more frequently, which is great exercise for my knee, ankle and the rest of me!

If you have endured futile attempts at weight loss only to achieve roller coaster results, and you want a comfortable ride to a healthy, slim body, I hope this book will encourage you. I'm not sure that I would have bought in to the Food Pyramid for weight loss a year ago. It is so far removed from my previous mindset and the many years of dieting and eating experiments, I'm just not sure that I would have ever tried this, except for the health aspects necessary to save Bob's very life. What I did accept was that the Pyramid would provide a roadmap for health, and I knew that a healthy body is not a fat one.

In response to my pleas for a prognosis for Bob's health, the hospital experts provided a common reply: "It's a long, slow process." We're learning exactly what that means. Nearly a year later we've seen amazing changes. Some feeling has returned, more to his left leg than his left arm. Bob is generally much calmer than he was during those first few months after the stroke and can now nap in the afternoon without the fear of being alone, stranded. He has a little more energy and is able to maneuver his wheelchair from room to room, usually with no assistance. We play card games believing that the mental stimulation aids in the repair of damaged brain cells.

The current second round of physical therapy is encouraging as Bob is much more involved. The healthy eating has produced positive results, and there have been times that the danger of deviating from it is apparent. Recently he was served a regular soft drink instead of the diet version. Thankfully, we've learned the signs of extreme blood sugar and were able to correct it with a small amount of insulin. There are still times that the fragility of his general health is obvious with spells of weakness, nausea and extreme changes in body temperature, blood pressure and blood sugar. But we do see vast improvements compared to the condition of his body immediately after the stroke and in the few months following. It's a long process, and we believe in the power of prayer.

Bob is now able to weigh in at the doctor's office, and we were surprised to learn that he has lost nearly 70 pounds since that fateful Friday the 13th. He looks healthy!

For me, the weight is over! Now on the right path, I gathered the nerve to try on my dress from the high school prom (see first picture by Bill Barley) and it *almost* works. This will be a benchmark for me, and I believe that the extra fluff will continue to disappear and I'll be able to zip that dress before long. This too, is a long process.

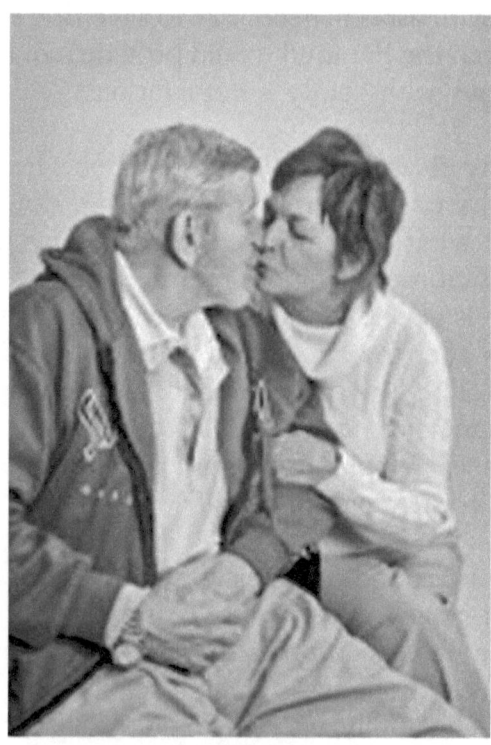

A year later

Chapter Seven

Thyroid Involvement
By Dr. Bob Galloway

I firmly believe that nothing happens by accident. There is always a reason. When this patient presented at my office with a neuro-musculoskeletal problem and started to describe the problems that her husband was having, the first thing that came to my mind was thyroid dysfunction.

Judi described the following symptoms: muscle and joint pain, weakness, fatigue, loss of memory, problems with concentration and depression. These are classic signs of hypothyroidism. Other symptoms might include goiter, drying skin with hair loss, loss of outer eyebrows, decreased reflexes, and high or low blood pressure. A properly functioning thyroid helps to prevent mental dulling, depression and memory loss.

I immediately recommended a thyroid panel to include TSH, T3, T4, and TPO antibody testing. This blood test is useful in ruling out primary hypothyroidism. When these tests come back abnormal, it is a sure sign that the patient is hypothyroid. The presence of TPO antibodies indicates Hashimoto's thyroiditis, which is an autoimmune disease that causes low thyroid output and can eventually lead to the destruction of the gland. However, many times patients have normal test results and are still presenting with the signs of hypothyroidism.

A physician should make the diagnosis from the patient history, the physical exam, and an evaluation of body temperature.

Hypothyroid-like symptoms that need to be differentially evaluated are:

(i) nutrient deficiencies such as zinc, selenium, the B vitamins and iodine;
(ii) estrogen dominance-induced hypothyroid symptoms; and
(iii) prolonged stress that affects the adrenal glands and can appear as hypothyroidism.

Primary hypothyroidism is currently medically treated with levothyroxine (Synthroid) (T4) or Armour thyroid (T4 & T3). But this is not always everything that needs to be done.

In my office I use a combination of testing to discover the root cause of these symptoms. A temperature test is performed by taking the basal body temperature for seven days. A temperature less than 97.5 may indicate an individual with a thyroid gland that is not functioning normally. I also suggest performing an iodine patch test. This test is performed by painting a one-inch square of iodine tincture on the wrist at the base of the hand. The brown color should disappear slowly after about 24 hours. If the color disappears too quickly, it may indicate the need for iodine and indicate sub-clinical hypothyroidism.

Iodine levels can also be more accurately evaluated using a provocative iodine loading test that is available from Hakala Research Reference Laboratory or FFP Laboratories. The patient is given a loading dose of iodine and urine output is collected over the next 24 hours. Depending on how much is excreted in the urine, a determination can be made as to the need of iodine. Treatment consists of a special combination of iodine and potassium iodide to restore normal levels. Iodine is required to make the enzyme that converts inactive T4 to T3.

It should also be understood that the thyroid gland is only one part of the patient's endocrine system. The brain and other glandular structures play a role in the normal functioning of the thyroid. The patient's overall health status should be evaluated. Key areas would include gastrointestinal function and liver detoxification, hormonal function and adrenal function.

Elevated estrogen levels can be evaluated in males and females using a saliva test. If estrogen is dominating, it can be controlled by dietary changes, herbals and hormone support when necessary. Adrenal function can also be evaluated with a saliva test that measures cortisol, DHEA and insulin levels. The appropriate adrenal support is determined and treated with DHEA, adrenal glandulars, herbals, vitamins and botanicals. Treatment usually requires between three weeks and three months of supplementation to reestablish normal levels of the nutrients that are required to restore normal function.

Hypothyroidism is a global problem. It is estimated that more than a third of the population of this country alone may be affected. Evaluation of this type of problem should include a skilled health professional who has experience with this functional problem and can lead a patient back to health.

Chapter Eight

Recipes

I'm not a chef and don't claim to be more than a loving cook for my family and friends. As you might have gathered, I do love good food and enjoy my own cooking. Following are some favorites, from daughter Marye and me.

Advice from daughter Niki, who is learning to be comfortable in the kitchen:

> Don't be afraid to store appliances like juicers, food processors and blenders on your counter tops (you can always remove them when company comes).

> Don't think that you must have everything in the store for food preparation – it's okay to improvise. (Although she gave me the most spectacular knives for Christmas, Niki is still happy enough with her own hand me downs.)

Advice from daughter Marye who loves to experiment and is very comfortable in the kitchen:

> There are some things you *must* have on hand:.
> Sesame oil (she prefers toasted)
> Extra Virgin Olive Oil (EVOO) – or just make sure it's "extra"
>   and not "light"

Citrus Grill Seasoning (Durkee brand) – the basic ingredients are
lemon peel, dill, garlic, onion, red bell pepper and paprika
Cavenders Greek Seasoning
Real butter – use exclusively
Sesame seeds to use in salads

All lemon/lime juice should be fresh squeezed
Mix EVOO and butter for sautéing – over medium-low heat
to prevent burning
Good music to cook and enjoy life by: Anything by Gabrielle
Roth and the Mirrors

Quick Chicken Soup

Such a healthy, tasty meal – easy to prepare. Use leftovers for lunch
and freeze remainder.

1 purchased roasted chicken and the drippings
1 can chicken stock or at least 4 cups homemade stock (recipe below)
½ large onion, chopped
2–3 large garlic cloves, chopped
1 inch ginger root, peeled and sliced
1 stalk celery with leaves
1 large turnip root, chopped
3-4 carrots chopped
2 bay leaves
1 tsp. tarragon
1 sprig fresh rosemary
Salt and pepper to taste
Garnish with grated cheese and sour cream

In a skillet, sauté chopped onion, garlic and ginger. Add to soup pot
and cover with canned chicken stock and water to total at least 2
quarts liquid. Add the celery stalk and leaves (remove before serving),
chopped carrots and turnip root.
I remove the legs and wings of the chicken for serving on the side or
as a protein serving at another meal.

Remove the skin and debone the chicken, chop the meat and add to the soup pot. Add any juices from the purchased roasted chicken.
Save all the skin and bones and set aside.
Add bay leaves, tarragon, rosemary, salt and pepper.
Bring soup to near boil, then reduce heat to low/medium and enjoy the aroma.
Once the carrots and turnip are tender, ladle servings into bowls and garnish with grated cheese and a dollop of sour cream. Add a sprig of parsley.

Serve with toasted tortillas. Cut in quarters; spread a small amount of butter (remember the fat requirements) and sprinkle with granulated garlic. Toast under the broiler on a cookie sheet.

Chicken stock for the next time

While the soup is cooking, add all the bones, skin (everything from the roasted chicken not used in the soup) to another soup pot. Cover with water and add chopped onion, garlic, carrots and celery. Bring to a near boil, then turn heat to low. When you're cleaning the kitchen after dinner, let the pot cool, and set it in the refrigerator. Begin cooking on low the next morning and continue all day, adding water as necessary. Cool completely and use a colander to strain, saving the liquid only. It freezes well and you're all set for the next soup, without using canned chicken stock, which is usually high in sodium.

Meatloaf

1-2 pounds ground beef or turkey
1 package onion soup mix
1 large egg
2 tbsp. Worcestershire Sauce
3 cup water

Put all ingredients in a bowl and mix thoroughly with your hands. Scoop and pat mixture into a lightly greased (baking sprays work well) loaf pan and bake at 425 for about an hour. I set the oven for 50 minutes and check then. When juices run clear, it's done.

Remove from oven to cool for at least 10 minutes before transferring to a platter for slicing.

Served with mashed white or sweet potatoes and corn or peas, it makes a healthy meal.

Leftover slices will keep in the refrigerator or freezer and make sandwiches or another meal.

Note: When using ground chicken, add fresh chopped parsley or cilantro and salsa or bruchetta.

Meatloaf option

Instead of making a loaf (or double the recipe and do both), prepare mixture into patties and cook at 350 degrees in an electric skillet. Brown quickly on both sides, cover and reduce heat. Remember, Rachel Ray says, "Resist the urge to press juice from the patties!" They'll be nice and moist.

Serve on whole-wheat buns with your favorite condiments.

The patties are easy to freeze alone or on buns. If you freeze on buns, remember to cool the patties completely first. Wrap each in foil and store in a tightly sealed freezer bag; meal prep will be easy the next time!

Marye's Meatloaf

1 pound ground turkey
1 cup crushed pretzels
1 egg
1 tsp. sesame oil
Greek seasoning to taste – at least 1 tsp.
Citrus grill seasoning – at least 1 tsp.
Chopped green onions and cilantro
2 tbsp. sesame seeds
¼ tsp. pepper and salt to taste

Mix and bake at 400 degrees for 45-60 minutes.

Bonus Meatloaf

1-2 pounds ground beef (or turkey)
Everything from a vegetable juicing – all the pulp, about 2-3 cups
2 tbsp. Worcestershire Sauce
2 packages onion soup mix
½ cup warm water
2 large eggs slightly beaten
Salt and pepper optional

Mix well and bake at 400 degrees for approximately 60 minutes, or until the juices run clear. Remove from oven and cool for 15-20 minutes, drain off juices and turn out on platter for slicing. The refrigerated slices make *wonderful* sandwiches. Bob prefers white bread (he gets white wheat) and I like heavy grainy bread. Try it, you'll love it!

Spaghetti Sauce – quick and easy

1-2 jars of sauce (look for the one with the least amount of sugar)
1 can diced tomatoes
1 small onion – peeled and chopped
3 large garlic cloves – peeled and chopped
1 sprig fresh rosemary
1 small bunch of fresh basil
3 bay leaves
1-2 stalks celery with leaves
3 cup red wine
1 cup water from cooked pasta
1 pound ground beef, turkey and/or sausage (I use left over cooked sweet Italian)
Salt and pepper to taste
1 tbsp. Italian seasoning
3 tbsp. dried parsley flakes and/or cilantro (if you're not using fresh)
1 tsp. tarragon

Empty jarred sauce and diced tomatoes in a large pot and turn on very low heat.
In a skillet, with 1-2 tbsp. of EVOO, sauté the chopped onion and garlic and add to sauce.

Brown the ground beef or turkey, adding salt and pepper. Drain well in a colander and add to sauce mixture.

Add celery with leaves and remove before serving.

Add parsley, tarragon, bay leaves and Italian seasoning.

Optional – add sliced sausage.

While this is cooking (the longer the better), add the red wine (optional) and prepare pasta.

When the pasta is done, ladle a cup of the water into the sauce and stir. Continue cooking on low, adding water if necessary.

Serve over pasta (look for whole wheat or other options to regular pasta).

Instead of pasta, I prefer the sauce served over sautéed zucchini squash. Wash and slice diagonally in one-inch pieces. Sauté in a skillet with EVOO, Italian seasoning, salt and pepper to taste.

Serve with whole wheat French bread sliced and toasted under the broiler. In a microwave bowl, place a half stick of butter with fresh chopped herbs (I like parsley and rosemary), chopped garlic, salt and pepper to taste and microwave 45 seconds or until the butter is melted. Pour or spread the mixture over the bread before toasting. Delicious!

Marye's Chick Pea Salad

1 large can garbanzo beans (drained and rinsed)
1 bunch green onions – green and white tops (chopped fine)
1 tbsp. sesame oil
Salt to taste
Citrus grill seasoning to taste
Juice of 1-2 limes
Mix the above, chill and enjoy

Marye's Own Portobello Mushroom with Spinach and Lime

1 portobello mushroom
1 "glop" of goat cheese (plain or basil – or your favorite)
1 huge handful of fresh spinach
1 large juicy lime
1 tbsp. EVOO and 1 tbsp. butter – twice
Greek seasoning to taste

Wipe mushroom and remove stem (save the stem for later).
Sautee mushroom cap in EVOO and butter until a little more tender than raw; flip and add goat cheese to the center of the mushroom cap.
Turn off heat, cover with tight lid.
In another skillet, add EVOO, Greek seasoning and fresh spinach; heat and cover until spinach is wilted (1-2 minutes).
Put wilted spinach on a plate and add the mushroom on top. Squeeze lime juice over all. Yum!

Marye's Tomato/Cucumber Salad

3 or 4 Roma tomatoes
1-2 cucumbers
Mozzarella or Monterey Jack cheese
Equal amounts of olive oil and red wine vinegar
½ tsp. salt
Lots of freshly ground black pepper – a tsp. at least

Cut tomatoes in quarters and squeeze out juice and seeds; dice into ½ inch pieces.
Peel cucumbers and cut lengthwise, scooping out seeds.
Dice cheese in ½ inch pieces.
Mix all ingredients and add about 5 counts of olive oil, 3-4 counts of vinegar and salt.
Add pepper until you can see it throughout the salad. Mix, taste and adjust to your liking.

Judi's Cookies

2 sticks butter, softened
½ cup firmly packed brown sugar
½ cup no-sugar-added applesauce
½ cup granulated sugar
½ cup Xylo Sweet (brand name for sugar substitute Xylitol)
2 eggs (room temperature)
1 tsp. vanilla extract
1-¾ cup flour* (I often use pastry wheat flour)
1 tsp. baking soda
1 tsp. cinnamon

½ tsp. salt
3 cups quick or old fashioned uncooked oatmeal
1 cup raisins, dates, dried apricots, a combination or any dried fruit(s)
1 cup semi-sweet chocolate chips
1-2 cups walnuts
½ cup coconut
*for high altitude, increase flour to 2 cups
Preheat oven to 350 degrees

Mix butter, applesauce, sugars and Xylo well in the food processor.
Add eggs and vanilla and process again.
Add walnuts and process for about 3 seconds to slightly chop.
In a large mixing bowl combine the flour, baking soda, cinnamon, salt, oatmeal, fruit(s), chocolate chips and coconut. Mix with a spatula or wooden spoon to evenly distribute, making sure all fruit is coated with the flour mixture.
Add mixture from the processor to the dry ingredients and stir by hand until the two are completely incorporated.

Cover cookie sheets with parchment paper.
Drop a spoonful of the mixture for each cookie and slightly flatten.
Bake 12-18 minutes until cookies are just turning golden.
Remove from oven and cool on cookie sheet for about 10 minutes.
Move carefully to finish cooling on a rack. If there are any left after the cooling, store in your favorite container. They freeze well.